BAKING WITH LESS SUGAR

RECIPES FOR DESSERTS USING LITTLE-TO-NO SUGAR

VALERIU COTET

VICI PUBLISHING

Copyright © 2015

TABLE OF CONTENTS

INTRODUCTION

Sugar is sugar. So it is yet is there any distinction in the kind of sugar that you and your family ingest? Truly, not by any stretch of the imagination. Your body really processes all sugar similarly yet the issue is that there is a great deal of sugar that is consolidated into every one of the nourishments we eat which puts a gigantic strain on the framework all in all.

Obviously, some say that the more common sugars, for example, fructose are less demanding to process and this may be valid since organic product when all is said in done is useful for your body yet every other sugar is exceptionally handled and accordingly would fall into a comparable classification as natural sweetener or corn sugar or syrup. At last, sugar will be sugar and your body must utilize insulin to separate sugar.

The American diet has seen an immense increment in sugar that is found in our day by day diet. Solace regards, for example, frozen yogurt and chocolate cake appear to be adding to the expansion of diabetes and hypoglycemia that is showing up at a more youthful age. Is it true that we are truly aware of the sugar content and the harm that these sugars are doing to our own wellbeing and the soundness of our general country?

It is really basic information that jams, jams and cremes have a high sugar content, however did you know nutty spread and most breads are sugar stacked also. These minimal known or publicized truths about the child sustenances we give our youngsters truly give them a weeks worth of sugar. These sustenances are considered non sweet nourishment things by the sponsors and fall into the same classification as wafers, breads and so on so we truly don't make the sugar association unless we instruct ourselves to what we are truly eating.

CUT THE SUGAR FROM YOUR DIET

Sugar from milk and natural product sources, for occurrence, ought not surpass 10% of aggregate kcalories. Concentrated refined sugars (e.g., table sugar) ought to be constrained however much as could be expected. The goal is to search for different names on nourishment bundling that are sugars, including corn syrup, dextrose, sucrose, corn sweeteners, glucose, fructose, lactose, nectar, molasses, maple sugar, maple syrup, sorbitol, mannitol, xylitol, maltose, or anything with "sugar" in the name, e.g., confectioner's sugar, or rearrange sugar.

The following step would be to lessen or supplant straightforward sugars with these proposals:

Lessen sugar in formulas. Indeed, even with a boundless diminishment of up to 20% or more, numerous formulas taste the same. With a few formulas a large portion of the sugar can be substituted with an equivalent bit of a sweet zest, for example, cinnamon, fennel, cardamom, allspice, anise, and ginger.

Numerous breakfast oats contain high rates of sugar. Search for those that don't have included sugar and best the oat with natural product if important and favored.

Substitute natural product juices for organic product drinks, soda pops, punches, and different fluids that contain high measures of sugar.

In the case of substituting sugars, know that there are two sorts of sweeteners or sugar substitutes. The main sort is a class of nutritive sweeteners that retain slower than sucrose, they don't advance dental caries, and they do contain kcalories. The second is a class of simulated sweeteners that don't contain kcalories, and they are alright for use for diabetics and calorie diminished eating methodologies.

Utilizing sugar substitutes (particularly counterfeit sweeteners) ought not give individuals permit to devour a lot of these items just in light of the fact that they are low in kcalories. They additionally have a tendency to be low in other supplement values and it is indistinct what restorative conditions can emerge from over-utilization. Consequently, these items ought not be a substitute for crisp natural products, vegetables, or different sustenances. Notwithstanding, on the off chance that it is hard to endure the day without a pudding, for instance, pick one made with skim milk and a sweetener than a high-fat, high-sugar sort.

Sugar Substitute Sweeteners

Nutritive Sweeteners
Fructose – Found in natural products, nectar, and some sweet vegetables. Fuctose ingests more gradually in the GI tract than glucose and metabolizes straightforwardly in the liver autonomous of insulin. Vast admissions of 70+ grams for each day can bring about looseness of the bowels.

Sorbitol – A sugar liquor discovered fundamentally in plants and utilized as a part of sweet shops (treat), gum, toothpaste, and diabetic pastries. After retention, sorbitol oxidizes into fructose. Sorbitol results in a slower, less maintained ascent in blood glucose than sugar. More than 10 grams for each day might bring about loose bowels.

Xylitol – A compound got from wood sugar. It causes minimal damage to teeth of every nutritive sweetener. Does not increment blood glucose levels. Admission of more than 30 grams for every day might bring about the runs. Additionally, it might be connected with bladder stones and tumors.

Counterfeit Sweeteners
Acesulfame K – An engineered sweetener that is exceptionally steady in warmth. Showcased as Sweet One, Sunette, or Sun Sweet Tabletop.

Aspartame – Best known as NutraSweet, it is discovered for the most part in sodas, gums, pudding blends, and different sustenances. It comprises of amino acids that separate in the GI tract, then it ingests and metabolizes. It has a low supplement and caloric worth.

Saccharin – Better known as Sweet'n Low, Nutra-eat less, and Sugar Twin, Saccharin is utilized basically as a part of soda pops and canned organic product. It neither metabolizes or stores in the body, yet discharges in the pee. Saccharin has a sharp persistent flavor, is low in kcalories , and may be a conceivable cancer-causing agent.

Sucralose – Available just in Canada to date. It contains no kcalories and is gotten from sugar. It is utilized as a part of cooking.

TIPS AND TRICKS

Making delightful sugar free and low sugar treats is currently less demanding than at any other time, because of another era of sugar free blends, frostings, chocolate and that's just the beginning.

Cutting sugar from your eating routine doesn't mean saying goodbye to an affectionate to sweet treats until the end of time. It's presently simpler than at any other time to make low and no sugar confections and pastries that are genuinely scrumptious by utilizing easy route fixings found as a part of most markets.

One of the coolest easy route fixings you can use to make sweet treats is canned sugar free icing. Both vanilla and chocolate assortments are accessible, and they make a great base for truffles, treat focuses, and cake pops. One of incredible elements of these frostings is you can warm them, which makes them tackle a fluid structure, and when they cool they come back to their past semi-firm state. This comes in exceptionally helpful for plunging natural products, sugar free treats, and sugar free cake or brownie squares.

While utilizing these frostings as a primary fixing in truffle focuses, it's a smart thought to consolidate them with somewhat dissolved sugar free chocolate. This makes the truffle more thick, firm, and simple to work with. Sugar free chocolate is presently accessible in the preparing path of most markets, and it not just melts and cooks precisely like conventional chocolate, additionally has a practically indistinguishable taste. You can utilize it in any formula as you would chocolate, including chocolate chip treats, plunged chocolates, and confection focuses. Since it liquefies precisely like chocolate does, you can likewise sprinkle it on a wide assortment of sugar free treats to make a delectable and alluring garnish.

Cake and brownie blends are additionally now accessible in sugar free assortments, which give important easy routes in low and no sugar formulas. These blends come in vanilla cake, fallen angels sustenance cake, and fudge brownie, and can be utilized anyplace a formula calls for such a blend. Cake blends are a continuous fixing in treat formulas, and such formulas are shamefully simple to make, as well as more often than not yield an entirely scrumptious treat. Attempt your most loved cake blend treat formulas utilizing a sugar free cake blend, and you'll see that the subsequent treats are unfathomably like the full sugar assortments.

Sugar free gelatin and pudding/pie filling blends are another useful standby in low and no sugar treat making. These blends additionally cook indistinguishably to the full sugar assortments, and taste for all intents and purposes the same. You can change your most loved Jello and pudding blend formulas to contain far less calories and practically zero sugar by utilizing these sugar free blends, with verging on indistinguishable tasting and looking results.

Sugar free and low sugar natural product pie fillings are another incredible alternate route fixing which can offer you some assistance with making fast, simple, and heavenly sugar free treats. Don't simply constrain these to pies; they make brilliant cake fillings, luscious waste of time layers, and can even be warmed up and utilized as a sweet, natural product topping for your most loved low sugar frozen yogurts.

It's imperative to eat these treats with some restraint. Despite the fact that they're sans sugar and contain far less calories than full sugar desserts, they're unquestionably not calorie free sustenances. Still, they're a perfect distinct option for full sugar sustenances for periodic treats. In the event that overabundance calories aren't sufficient of a motivator to relax with these sugar free alternate way nourishments, there's another squeezing reason - maltitol. Maltitol is a sweetener which loans richness and surface to nourishments, and is the primary fixing in sugar free chocolate and icing. In the event that eaten exorbitantly, it can bring about gastric miracle. Restricting yourself to little , infrequent servings of maltitol-rich nourishments ought to keep any undesirable reactions.

CHOCOLATE CAKE

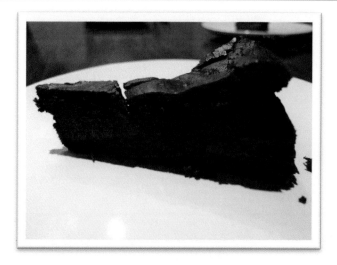

INGREDIENTS

- 75g cocoa powder
- 125g caster sugar
- 3 tsp vanilla extract
- 50ml walnut oil
- 1 large egg
- 225g plain flour
- 21 tsp baking powder

INSTRUCTIONS

1. Drain the pears, reserving the juice. Measure the cocoa, sugar and 125ml of pear juice into a saucepan, madly whisk it all together and bring to the first plop of a boil.
2. Spoon this mixture, along with the pear halves, into a mixing bowl and leave to cool for 15 minutes.
3. Line the bottom and sides of a 20cm round cake tin with non-stick baking paper and preheat the oven to 170C.

Spoon the chocolate mixture, vanilla and oil into a blender, and purée until smooth.

4. Pour this back into the bowl, then beat in the egg. Stir together the flour and baking powder, sift into the bowl and beat until smooth.

5. Scrape the mixture into the cake tin and bake for 40 minutes.

BANANA CAKE

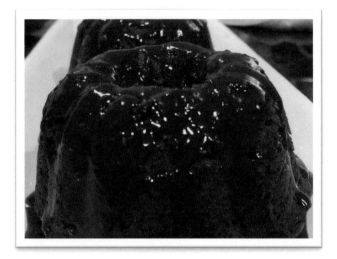

INGREDIENTS

Cake

- 2 cups all-purpose flour
- ½ cup whole wheat pastry flour
- ½ cup granulated sugar
- ½ cup packed brown sugar
- 1 ¼ teaspoons baking powder
- 1 teaspoon ground cinnamon

- ½ teaspoon salt
- ½ teaspoon baking soda
- ¾ cup fat-free milk
- ½ cup refrigerated or frozen egg product, thawed, or 2 eggs, lightly beaten
- 2/3 cup mashed banana
- ¼ cup canola oil
- 1 teaspoon vanilla

GANACHE

- 3 ounces dark chocolate, chopped
- ¼ cup fat-free half-and-half

INSTRUCTIONS

CAKE

1. Preheat oven to 325 degrees F. Generously grease and flour a 10-inch fluted tube pan; set pan aside. In large mixing bowl stir together flours, granulated and brown sugar, baking powder, cinnamon, salt, and baking soda.
2. In medium bowl combine milk, eggs, banana, oil, and vanilla. Add egg mixture all at once to flour mixture. Beat with an electric mixer on medium to high speed for 2 minutes. Spoon batter into prepared pan; spread evenly.
3. Bake about 45 to 55 minutes. Cool in pan on a wire rack for 10 minutes. Remove the cake from pan. Cool completely on a wire rack.

GANACHE

1. In a small microwave-safe bowl combine chocolate and half-and-half. Microwave, uncovered, on 50% power (medium) for 1 minute.
2. Let it stand for 5 minutes. Stir until completely smooth. Let it stand to thicken slightly. Spoon evenly atop cooled cake.

CAKE ROLL

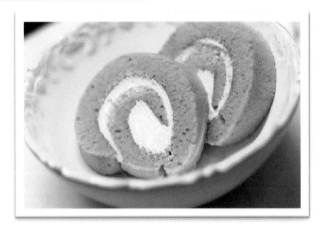

Ingredients

- 4 eggs
- 1/3 cup all-purpose flour
- 1 tablespoon unsweetened cocoa powder
- 1 teaspoon baking powder
- ½ teaspoon vanilla
- 1/3 cup granulated sugar
- 1 tablespoon red food coloring
- ½ cup granulated sugar
- powdered sugar
- 1 cup frozen light whipped dessert topping, thawed
- ½ cup light sour cream
- ½ teaspoon vanilla

INSTRUCTIONS

1. Separate eggs. Allow egg whites and yolks to stand at room temperature 30 minutes.
2. Grease a 15x10x1-inch baking pan. Line bottom of pan with waxed paper or parchment paper; grease paper. Set

pan aside. In a medium bowl stir together flour, cocoa powder, and baking powder.

3. Preheat the oven to 375 degrees F. In a medium bowl beat egg yolks and ½ teaspoon vanilla with a mixer on high speed about 5 minutes. Gradually add the 1/3 cup granulated sugar, beating on high speed until sugar is almost dissolved. Beat in the food coloring.

4. Thoroughly wash beaters. In another medium bowl beat egg whites on medium speed until soft peaks form. Gradually add the ½ cup granulated sugar, beating until stiff peaks form. Fold egg yolk mixture into beaten egg whites. Sprinkle flour mixture over egg mixture; gently fold in just until combined. Spread batter evenly in the prepared baking pan.

5. Bake 12 to 15 minutes. Immediately loosen edges of cake from pan and turn cake out onto a clean kitchen towel sprinkled with powdered sugar. Remove waxed paper. Starting from a short side, roll up towel and cake into a spiral. Cool on a wire rack.

FILLING

1. In a medium bowl fold together dessert topping, sour cream, and ½ teaspoon vanilla. Unroll cake; remove towel.

2. Spread the cake with filling to within 1 inch of the edges. Roll up cake into a spiral; trim ends. Cover and chill up to 6 hours. Just before serving, sprinkle cake with additional powdered sugar.

BANANA BREAD WITH CHOCOLATE

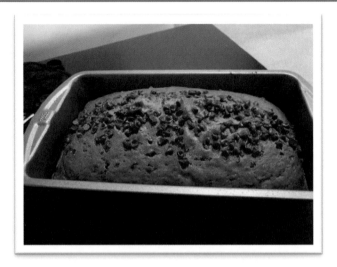

INGREDIENTS

- 2 cups overripe mashed banana, loosely packed
- 2 ½ tsp pure vanilla extract
- 1 tbsp vinegar
- ¼ cup oil
- 2/3 cup pure maple syrup or agave
- ¼ cup sugar
- 1 ¾ flour
- 1 tsp baking soda
- ¾ tsp salt
- ¾ tsp baking powder
- ½ cup plus 2 tbsp cocoa powder
- ½ cup mini chocolate chips in the batter

INSTRUCTIONS

1. Preheat oven to 350 F and grease a 9×5 loaf pan very well. In a large mixing bowl, whisk together first six ingredients.

2. In a separate bowl, combine all remaining ingredients and stir well. Pour dry into wet, and stir until just evenly combined. Transfer to the loaf pan and spread out evenly.
3. Bake 35 minutes, then turn off the oven and don't open the door! Let sit 10 additional minutes in the closed oven before removing and slicing. This tastes even sweeter the next day.

APPLESAUCE BROWNIES

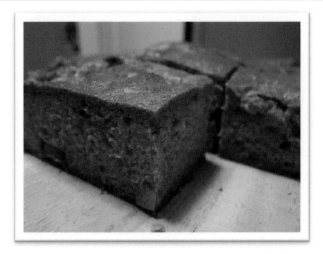

INGREDIENTS

- ½ cup coconut flour, sifted
- ¾ cup unsweetened applesauce
- ½ cup coconut palm sugar
- ½ cup nut butter of choice
- cinnamon, for dusting

INSTRUCTIONS

1. Line a small baking tray with baking paper and set aside.

2. In a mixing bowl, combine your coconut flour and coconut palm sugar and mix well. Add your applesauce and nut butter and mix until a very thick batter is formed.
3. Transfer the batter to the lined baking tray, top with extra cinnamon and sugar and refrigerate for an hour or so, until it has firmed up slightly.

LOW-SUGAR BARS

INGREDIENTS

- 100g plain flour
- 100g plain wholemeal flour
- 1 tsp baking powder
- 1 tsp ground mixed spice
- 225g sultanas
- 175g barley malt extract
- 2 tbsp honey
- 2 large eggs, lightly beaten
- 150ml cold black tea

INSTRUCTIONS

1. Preheat the oven to 150C, gas 2. Place greaseproof mini loaf cases onto a baking tray.
2. Weigh the plain flour, wholemeal flour, baking powder, mixed spice and sultanas into a large mixing bowl.
3. Add the malt extract and the honey into a small saucepan and place over a low heat. As soon as the mixture becomes runny, take it off the heat.
4. Pour the cold black tea, beaten eggs and malt mixture into the bowl of dry ingredients. Use a wooden spoon and mix to combine.
5. Spoon the mixture into the mini loaf tins and fill ¾ of cases.

6. Place your malt loaves into the pre-heated oven and leave to cook. Bake until a skewer inserted into the middle of the loaf, comes out clean.
7. Leave the malt loaves to cool in the tin for around 10 minutes and then turn out to cool completely on a wire rack.
8. Leave them overnight.

BUNDT CAKE

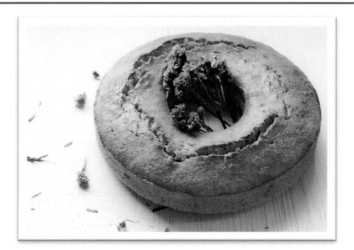

INGREDIENTS

- 240g gluten-free flour
- 31tsps baking powder
- 1tsp ground cinnamon
- 1tsp salt
- 475ml unsweetened apple purée/applesauce
- 120ml agave syrup or pure maple syrup
- 80ml rice milk
- 75g golden raisins

INSTRUCTIONS

1. Preheat the oven to 180°C/350°F/Gas mark 4. Sift the flour and baking powder together into a bowl, then add the cinnamon and salt and mix by hand.
2. Create a hole or a well in the centre of the ingredients. Separately, combine the apple purée/applesauce, agave syrup and rice milk.
3. Pour this wet mixture, one third at a time, into the well in your bowl of dry ingredients. Stir as you go. Be sure not to overmix. Add the dried fruit and make sure it is well distributed throughout the mixture.
4. Spoon the mixture into the baking pan. Bake in the middle of the preheated oven for 40 minutes.
5. Allow the cake to cool for at least 10 minutes before cutting into it.

CIFFON CAKE

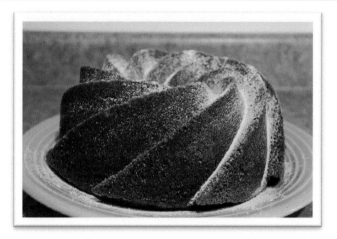

INGREDIENTS

- 6 egg whites
- 4 egg yolks
- ¾ cup cubed cantaloupe
- ¾ cup sparkling white wine
- 8 cups cantaloupe, honeydew, and/or watermelon balls
- 1 2/3 cups cake flour
- 2/3 cup granulated sugar
- 2 teaspoons baking powder
- ¼ teaspoon salt
- ¼ teaspoon ground allspice
- 1/3 cup canola oil
- ¼ teaspoon cream of tartar
- powdered sugar
- 1 8 - ounce container frozen light whipped dessert topping, thawed

INSTRUCTIONS

3. Allow egg whites and yolks to stand at room temperature for 30 minutes. In a blender, combine the ¾ cup cantaloupe and 2 tablespoons of the sparkling wine. Cover and blend until smooth. Set aside. Grease and lightly flour a 10-inch fluted tube pan; set aside.
4. In a large bowl, combine the remaining sparkling wine and the 8 cups cantaloupe. Toss gently to coat. Cover and chill until ready to serve.
5. Preheat oven to 325 degrees F. In a large bowl, combine cake flour, granulated sugar, baking powder, salt, and allspice. Make a well in the center of the flour mixture.
6. Add egg yolks, pureed cantaloupe mixture, and oil to flour mixture. Beat with an electric mixer on low speed until combined. Beat on high speed about 5 minutes more.
7. Wash beaters thoroughly with soap and warm water; dry beaters. In a very large bowl, combine egg whites and cream of tartar; beat with a mixer on medium speed until stiff peaks. Pour egg yolk mixture in a thin stream over beaten egg whites, folding gently as you pour. Pour into prepared pan and spread evenly.
8. Bake for 45 to 50 minutes.
9. Immediately invert cake in pan and cool completely. Loosen sides of cake from pan; remove cake. Place cake on a serving plate. If desired, sprinkle with powdered sugar and garnish with fresh

SNACK CAKE

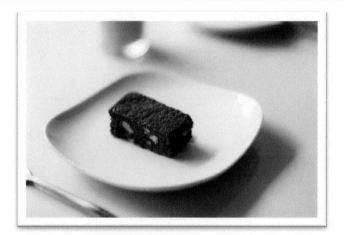

INGREDIENTS

- ¾ cup whole wheat flour
- ¾ cup flour
- 1 teaspoon baking soda
- ¼ cup cocoa
- 1/2 teaspoon salt
- 1 cup water
- ¼ cup applesauce
- 1 teaspoon lemon juice
- 1 teaspoon vanilla
- 1 apple, chopped and peeled
- ½ cup sugar
- ½ teaspoon cinnamon

INSTRUCTIONS

1. Oven to 350°.
2. Spray a square pan with nonstick spray.
3. Combine first 5 ingredients in bowl.
4. In another bowl, combine water, oil, lemon juice, vanilla.

5. Add to dry ingredients, stir until just combined.
6. Toss apples with sugar and cinnamon, fold into batter.
7. Pour into prepared pan.
8. Bake for 30-35 minutes or until done.

CARROT CAKE

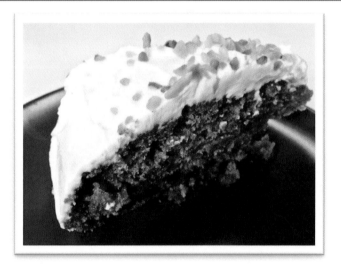

INGREDIENTS

- 1 ½ cup all-purpose flour
- 1/4 cup whole wheat flour
- 1 tsp. baking powder
- ½ tsp. baking soda
- ½ tsp. cinnamon
- ½ tsp. ginger
- ¼ tsp. salt
- ½ c. vegetable oil
- 6 tbsp. sugar
- 2 eggs

- ¼ c. unsweetened pineapple juice concentrate
- 1 tsp. vanilla
- 1 cup shredded carrots
- ½ cup golden raisins
- ½ cup crushed unsweetened pineapple, drained

FROSTING

1 8 oz. pkg. cream cheese
5 tbsp. unsweetened pineapple juice concentrate
½ tsp. vanilla
½ tsp. finely grated orange zest

INSTRUCTIONS

1. Preheat oven to 350°F. Grease and flour 9x5x3 inch pan.
2. In a bowl, toss dry ingredients. In second bowl, stir oil, sugar, eggs, juice and vanilla. Stir liquid into dry ingredients until smooth. Stir in carrots, raisins and pineapple. Scrape into prepared pan. Bake 35-40 minutes. Cool in pan on rack, 1 hour.
3. Unmold and ice with frosting.

FROSTING

Beat all ingredients together until smooth.

CHOCOLATE CAKE FLOUR-FREE

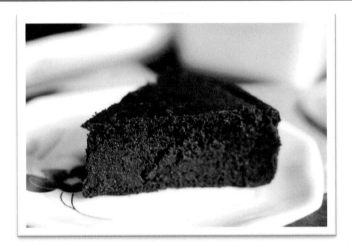

INGREDIENTS

- 4 oz. unsweetened baking chocolate
- 3 whole eggs
- ½ cup grass-fed butter, or coconut oil
- ¼ cup cocoa powder
- ¾ cup honey

INSTRUCTIONS

1. Preheat the oven to 375F, and grease an 8" spring-form pan generously with coconut oil or butter.
2. Melt the baking chocolate and butter together, stirring until completely smooth.
3. Combine the melted chocolate/butter with the cocoa powder, honey, and eggs, then whisk well until a smooth batter forms.
4. Pour the batter into the greased pan, and smooth the top with a spatula.

5. Bake at 375F for 20-25 minutes, until the center looks firm. Allow to cool in the pan for 15 minutes, then remove the sides and allow to cool completely before serving.

GOAT CHEESE FROSTING CAKE

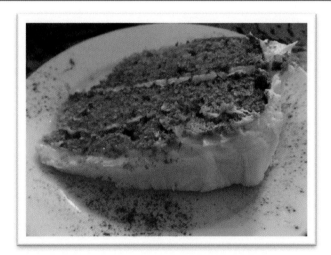

INGREDIENTS

CAKE

- 2 ½ cups unbleached all-purpose flour
- 3 teaspoons baking powder
- 1 ½ teaspoon baking soda
- 1/2 teaspoon cinnamon
- ¼ teaspoon salt
- 1 1/3 cup grated carrots
- 1 cup grated zucchini
- 1 cup finely grated beets
- ¾ cup chopped walnuts
- ½ cup raisins

- 1 1/3 cup pure maple syrup
- 2/3 cup safflower, canola or other mild-tasting oil
- 4 eggs

FROSTING

- 15 ounces fresh goat cheese, at room temperature
- 6 ounces cream cheese, room temperature
- 1 ½ cup powdered sugar
- 1 cup pure maple syrup

GARNISH

- 8-12 walnut halves or ½ cup finely chopped walnuts
- flowers

INSTRUCTIONS

1. Arrange oven racks to divide oven into thirds. Preheat oven to 400° F Grease two 9in x 2in cake pans, dust with a spoonful of flour and tap out. Line each with a round of parchment paper.
2. Sift together flour, baking powder, baking soda, cinnamon and salt into a bowl. In another bowl, stir together carrots, zucchini, beets, nuts, and raisins.
3. In a large mixing bowl, beat maple syrup and oil together until emulsified. Add eggs one at a time, beating until batter is smooth. Add flour mixture in three or four batches, mixing gently until mixture is even. Gently mix in the vegetable mixture. Divide between baking pans.
4. Place one baking pan in center of each of the racks. Bake for 25-35 minutes. Cool on a rack for about 5 minutes, then gently remove from pans. Cool to room temperature before frosting.

FROSTING

1. Using an electric mixer or a wooden spoon and a strong arm, beat goat cheese and cream cheese together until light and fluffy.
2. Add powdered sugar and beat at low speed until well blended. Beat in maple syrup. Chill about 30 minutes.

1. Cut four strips of parchment or wax paper to line cake plate under the cake's edges.
2. Place first cake layer on plate. Using an off-set spatula or table knife, spread with frosting, pushing it to edges. Place second layer, top down, squarely on first layer.
3. Spread a thin layer of frosting over entire cake to eliminate crumbs. Frost with remaining frosting. Arrange walnut halves and/or flowers around edge.

PANCAKES

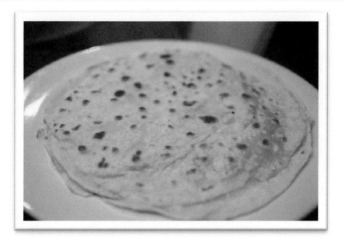

INGREDIENTS

- 3 medium eggs
- 25g runny honey
- 150ml ale or bitter
- 150g double cream
- 100g plain flour
- 25g wheatgerm
- 1 pinch of salt

- butter, for frying

INSTRUCTIONS

1. Whisk the eggs in a bowl. Beat in the honey, ale and cream, add the flour, wheatgerm and salt, and beat smooth.
2. Melt half a teaspoon of butter in a frying pan. Pour in enough batter lightly to cover the surface and cook until the surface sets and the edges start to brown.
3. Use a spatula to loosen the pancake, flip and cook the other side. Keep warm, and repeat with the remaining batter.

CHOCOLATE FUDGE

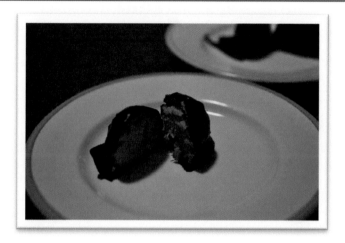

INGREDIENTS

FILLING

- one batch peanut butter fudge

SHELL

- 4oz dark chocolate, chopped into chunks
- 1 tsp coconut oil

PEANUT BUTTER FUDGE

- ½ cup peanut butter or allergy-friendly alternative (110g)
- 1 large banana (150g)
- 1 tsp pure vanilla extract
- pinch of salt
- 2 tbsp coconut butter
- 2 tbsp powdered sugar

Instructions

PEANUT BUTTER FUDGE

1. Either combine all ingredients in a small blender until completely smooth or mash the banana and stir together ingredients very patiently by hand until completely smooth.
2. Scoop into a small plastic container. Freeze until firm.

SHELLS AND ASSEMBLY

1. After refrigerating overnight and slicing the fudge, place the fudge cubes on a cookie tray lined with a sheet of parchment paper. Place in the refrigerator while you prepare the chocolate.
2. In a microwave-safe bowl, add the chocolate and microwave at 30-second intervals, stirring between each one, until melted, then stir in the coconut oil.
3. Take the fudge out of the fridge. Toss a piece of fudge into the chocolate and use a fork to coat it entirely and remove it from the chocolate. Tap off any excess chocolate, then place the cube onto the prepared cookie sheet. Do this with the rest of the fudge, and reheat the chocolate if necessary.
4. Chill the cubes until the chocolate hardens, then serve.

BROWNIES

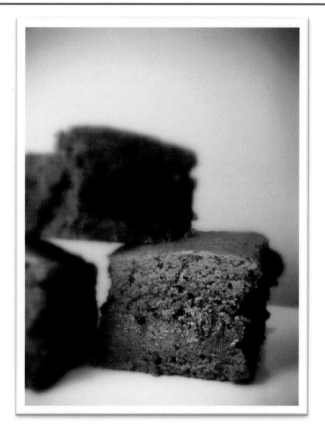

INGREDIENTS

- ¾ cup nonfat Greek yogurt
- ¼ cup skim milk
- ½ cup cocoa powder
- ½ cup old fashioned rolled oats
- ½ cup stevia in the raw (or coconut sugar)
- 1 egg
- 1/3 cup applesauce (unsweetened)
- 1 teaspoon baking powder

- 1 pinch salt

1. Preheat the oven to 400°F. Grease a square baking dish . Combine all ingredients into a food processor or a blender, and blend until smooth.
2. Pour into the prepared dish and bake for about 15 minutes. Allow to cool completely before cutting.

BANANA BREAD

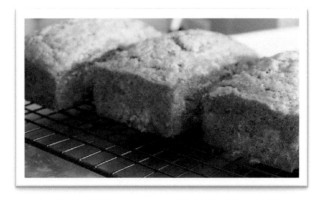

INGREDIENTS

- 1 cup + 1 tbsp ripe mashed banana
- 2 ½ tbsp honey
- 2 tsp vanilla extract
- 3 ½ tbsp butter or coconut oil, melted
- ¼ cup unsweetened applesauce
- 4 eggs
- ½ cup coconut flour
- ½ cup almond meal
- ¾ tsp baking soda

1. Preheat the oven to 170C/340F.
2. Grease and line a small loaf tin and set aside.
3. In a medium mixing bowl, mash the bananas and add in the honey, vanilla, melted butter/coconut oil, applesauce and eggs.
4. Mix in the coconut flour, baking soda and almond meal and allow to sit for two minutes.
5. Pour the banana bread mixture into the prepared loaf tin and bake for 40 minutes to an hour.
6. Allow to cool completely before slicing.

PEANUT BUTTER MUFFINS

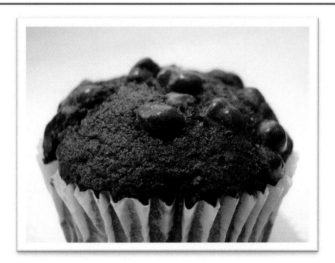

INGREDIENTS

- ¼ cup cocoa powder
- 2 tablespoons oat flour
- ½ teaspoon baking soda
- ¼ teaspoon baking powder

- ¼ teaspoon salt
- 2 tablespoons brown sugar, lightly packed
- ½ cup creamy peanut butter
- ¼ cup unsweetened applesauce
- ¼ cup plain Greek yogurt
- 1 teaspoon vanilla extract
- 2 tablespoons honey
- 1 large egg
- 5 tablespoons dark chocolate chips

INSTRUCTIONS

1. Preheat the oven to 425 degrees F. Spray the 9 of the cavities in a muffin tin and fill the other three up halfway with water.
2. In a large bowl, stir together the cocoa powder, oat flour, baking soda, baking powder, salt, and brown sugar.
3. In a separate bowl, combine the peanut butter, applesauce, Greek yogurt, vanilla, and honey. Beat until completely combined.
4. Beat together dry and wet ingredients and add in the egg.
5. Stir in the chocolate chips and top each muffin with a few more.
6. Bake at 425 degrees for 5 minutes and then reduce the heat to 350 degrees and continue to bake for 13-15 more minutes.

PUMPKIN MOUSSE

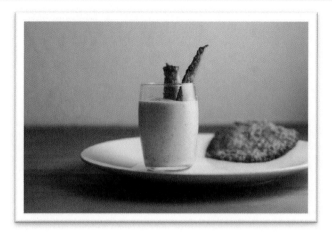

INGREDIENTS

- 2- 8 ounces packages cream cheese
  - 15 ounce can pure pumpkin puree
- 2 cups heavy cream
- pinch salt
- 2 teaspoons pumpkin pie spice
- 1-2 teaspoons vanilla liquid stevia or to taste
- 1 teaspoon vanilla extract

INSTRUCTIONS

1. In a stand mixer blend cream cheese and pumpkin until smooth.
2. Add the rest of the ingredients and blend until whipped and fluffy about 5 minutes.
3. Taste and adjust sweetener to your liking.
4. Pipe into serving glasses and top with cacao nibs or brown sugar(optional).
5. Keep refrigerated until ready to serve.

LEMON CAKE

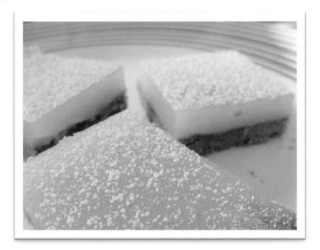

INGREDIENTS

CRUST

- 1-1/3 cup rolled oats
- ¼ cup unsweetened shredded coconut
- 7 dates
- ¾ tsp sea salt
- ¼ cup almond meal or almond flour
- ¼ cup coconut oil, melted

CREAM

- 2 cups coconut milk
- 2 Tbs agar agar flakes
- ¼ cup fresh lemon juice
- ¼ tsp lemon zest
- 3 Tbs + 1 tsp agave syrup
- ¼ tsp vanilla extract
- 3 pinches of turmeric

- 1 pinch of salt
- 6oz non-dairy plain yogurt

INSTRUCTIONS

1. Preheat oven to 350 degrees. Spray a 8 x 8 non-stick square cake pan with cooking spray.
2. Place the oats, shredded coconut, dates, and salt into a food processor and process for a minute or two until everything is flour-like consistency.
3. Add the almond meal and pulse 4 to 5 times to combine. Add the coconut oil and pulse until it just starts to come together as a dough. Sprinkle the mixture evenly into the prepared pan.
4. Use your fingers to gently press the crust down, leveling as needed. Transfer to the oven. Bake for 10-15 minutes. Set pan on a wire rack to cool to room temperature.
5. When crust has cooled, place the 2 cups of coconut milk into a medium saucepan and sprinkle the agar flakes on top. Let sit for a few minutes then add the lemon juice, zest, agave, vanilla, turmeric, and salt. Whisk to combine. Bring the mixture to a slow boil. Once the mixture comes to a rolling boil, set a timer for 10 minutes. Reduce the heat a bit (medium-low), and let the mix boil for 10 minutes, whisking frequently. After 10 minutes remove from heat and whisk in the yogurt. Pour this mixture carefully over the top of the cooled crust and place the pan in the fridge to set.

LAVA CAKE

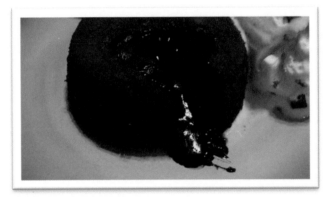

INGREDIENTS

- 4 oz semisweet or bittersweet chocolate
- 4 tablespoons extra virgin coconut oil
- 2 eggs
- ½ teaspoon vanilla extract
- 1/8 teaspoon salt
- 2 tablespoons sugar
- 2 teaspoons cocoa powder
- 1 teaspoon coconut flour

INSTRUCTIONS

1. Preheat oven to 375F. Grease four 6oz ramekins with coconut oil. Melt chocolate and coconut oil over low heat or a double boiler. Stir until smooth and let cool.
2. In a small bowl, beat eggs, vanilla, salt and sugar with a hand mixer until light and frothy, five minutes.
3. Pour the egg mixture over chocolate. Sift cocoa and coconut flour over the top. Then gently fold all the ingredients together.

4. Pour batter into prepared ramekins. Place the ramekins on a baking sheet and place in the oven. Bake for 11-12 minutes.
5. Remove from oven and serve immediately.

PUMPKIN DONUTS

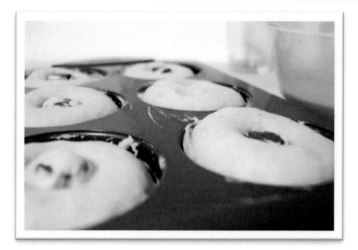

INGREDIENTS

- 1 box of yellow cake mix
- 1 can of pumpkin

INSTRUCTIONS

1. Heat oven to 400 degrees. Mix the dry cake mix (do not add oil, eggs, or water indicated on the back of the box) and can of pumpkin.
2. Fill each pan cavity ½ full. Bake for 8-10 minutes. Cool donuts completely before adding a caramel drizzle and/or powdered sugar. Eat immediately.

CHOCOLATE CAKE ON SLOW

COOKER

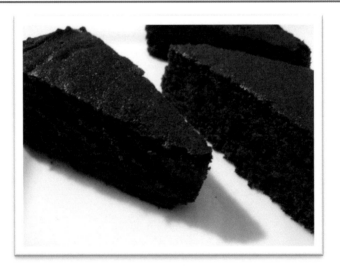

INGREDIENTS

- 1 ½ cups almond flour
- ¾ cup swerve sweetener
- 2/3 cup cocoa powder
- ¼ cup unflavoured whey protein powder
- 2 tsp baking powder
- ¼ tsp salt
- ½ cup butter, melted
- 4 large eggs
- ¾ cup almond or coconut milk, unsweetened
- 1 tsp vanilla extract
- ½ cup sugar-free chocolate chips

INSTRUCTIONS

1. Grease the insert of a 6 quart slow cooker well.
2. In a medium bowl, whisk together almond flour, sweetener, cocoa powder, whey protein powder, baking powder and salt.
3. Stir in butter, eggs, almond milk and vanilla extract until well combined, then stir in chocolate chips.
4. Pour into prepared insert and cook on low for 2 ½ to 3 hours. It will be gooey and like a pudding cake at 2 ½ hours, and more cakey at 3 hours.
5. Turn slow cooker off and let cool 20 to 30 minutes, then cut into pieces and serve warm.

CRUMBLE CAKE

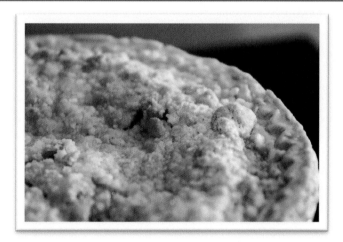

INGREDIENTS

- vegetable cooking spray
- 1 cup all-purpose flour
- 1/3 cup rolled oats
- 1/3 cup one-to-one sugar substitute
- ¼ cup brown sugar substitute
- 1 teaspoon ground cinnamon

- 1/8 teaspoon ground nutmeg
- 1/8 teaspoon salt
- 4 tablespoons cold margarine, cut into small pieces
- ½ teaspoon baking powder
- ½ teaspoon baking soda
- 1/3 cup unsweetened apple juice
- 1 teaspoon vanilla extract
- ¼ cup egg substitute
- 2 Braeburn apples, about 1 pound total, peeled, cored, and chopped

INSTRUCTIONS

1. Preheat the oven to 350° F. Lightly coat an 8-inch square baking pan with cooking spray.
2. In a bowl combine the flour, oats, sugar substitutes, cinnamon, nutmeg, and salt. Cut in the margarine with a pastry blender until the mixture looks like coarse meal. Set aside ½ cup.
3. Combine the remaining flour mixture with the baking powder, baking soda, apple juice, vanilla, and egg substitute. Beat at a medium speed with an electric mixture until blended. Fold in the apples.
4. Spoon the cake mixture into the pan and level out. Sprinkle with the reserved flour mixture. Bake for 30 to 35 minutes until the cake springs back in the center when lightly touched. Cool the cake until warm. Cut into 16 squares. Serve warm or cooled.

LOW-SUGAR BROWNIES

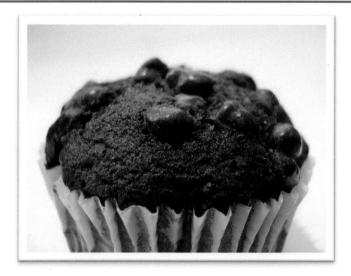

INGREDIENTS

- 1 can organic black beans
- 2 free run large eggs
- 3 Tbsp organic coconut oil, melted
- 5 Tbsp 100% cocoa
- 2 tsp baking powder
- ½ tsp baking soda
- ¼ tsp fine sea salt
- 3 Tbsp sweetener of choice
- 1 Tbsp maple or vanilla extract
- ½ cup chopped nuts

INSTRUCTIONS

1. Preheat oven to 350 degrees.
2. Rinse and drain beans.

3. Mix all ingredients, except nuts, together in mixing bowl, blender or food processor. Add nuts (except 1 Tbsp) and gently fold in.
4. Separate mixture into 12 lined muffin tins.
5. Top with left over nuts. Bake for about 22 minutes.

LOW SUGAR LEMON CHEESECAKE

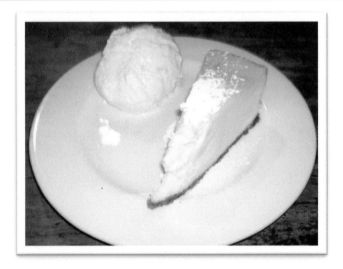

INGREDIENTS

CRUST

- 1¼ cup almond flour
- 3 tablespoons butter, melted
- 1½ teaspoon sweetener

FILLING

- 8 ounce cream cheese, softened
- ½ teaspoon vanilla extract
- 1½ cups heavy whipping cream

- 3 ounce packet sugar-free lemon jello

INSTRUCTIONS

CRUST

- Preheat oven to 350 degrees. Generously spray an 8-inch baking dish or springform pan with cooking spray.
- Mix almond flour, butter and splenda until mixture is crumbly. Press in the bottom of baking dish and bake for about 8-10 minutes.
- Cool completely.

FILLING

1. Using an electric mixer with the whisk attachment mix cream cheese until smooth and creamy.
2. Stir in vanilla extract.
3. Add in heavy cream and whisk on high until mixture thickens and soft peaks form.
4. Reduce speed to low and mix in jello packet until blended. Spread themixture evenly with a spatula over cooled crust.
5. Cover and chill until set, about 2-3 hours.

LAST WORDS...

I am glad that you stayed till the end of this book. If you've enjoyed reading this book and if you have found it useful, I would like to hear your feedback by writing a review or mailing me at cotetvaleriu@gmail.com

Thank you for your support and don't forget that you are AWESOME.

13388723R00029

Printed in Poland
by Amazon Fulfillment
Poland Sp. z o.o., Wrocław